THE
OBESITY FIGHTING
COOKBOOK

Healthy Recipes For

Permanent Weight Loss

By

Mary J. Douglas

Table of Contents

Introduction

Natasha Martins had been struggling with her weight for years. She was always the biggest person in the room and felt like she didn't fit in. She had tried every diet out there, but nothing seemed to work for her.

One day, a friend of hers introduced her to me and I gave her a copy of this cookbook for weight loss. She took it and suggested she give it a try, and she decided it was worth a shot.

It listed recipes for healthy breakfast, lunch, dinner, snacks, and desserts. She was excited to try something new and hopeful that this time would be different.

Over the next few weeks, Natasha followed the recipes in the book and made sure to stick to her new meal plan. She was surprised to find that she was starting to lose weight and feeling better than she had in a long time.

She kept up with her new eating habits and eventually reached her goal weight. She was so proud of herself and knew that she had finally found the right diet for her.

Natasha was so grateful to have found this cookbook and to have finally been able to reach her weight loss goals. She was no longer the biggest person in the room and was proud to show off her new figure. She was now able to enjoy life to the fullest and was thankful for the cookbook that had helped her get there.

Obesity has become an epidemic in our society, affecting individuals of all ages and backgrounds. It is a serious medical condition that can lead to a wide range of health issues, including diabetes, heart disease, stroke, and certain types of cancer. While there is no single solution to the problem of obesity, making healthy lifestyle changes and maintaining a balanced diet are essential steps to take. This cookbook is designed to help you achieve your health and weight loss goals by providing you with delicious and nutritious recipes that are low in calories and fat, yet still full of flavor. From vegetarian options to heart-healthy dishes, you'll find something to satisfy every palate and dietary need. With these recipes, you can enjoy delicious meals that will help you maintain a healthy weight and stay on track with your health goals.

Chapter 1

Understanding Obesity

Obesity is a complex, chronic health condition that is caused by an imbalance between energy consumed and energy expended. It is identified by an excess buildup of body fat. Obesity has many causes, including genetics, lifestyle, and environmental factors.

The most common cause of obesity is an imbalance between the amount of food consumed and the amount of physical activity. Eating too much and not exercising enough can lead to an increase in body fat, which can eventually lead to obesity. In addition, certain genetic and environmental factors can increase the risk of obesity, such as a family history of obesity, living in a food-insecure environment, or having a sedentary lifestyle.

Obesity can have serious health consequences, such as increased risk of type 2 diabetes, heart disease, stroke, certain types of cancer, and mental health issues. It is important to understand the causes of obesity in order to prevent and manage it. This includes maintaining a healthy diet, engaging in regular physical activity, and making lifestyle changes such as reducing stress and getting enough sleep.

In addition to diet and exercise, there are a variety of treatments available to those who are living with obesity, such as medications, bariatric surgery, and lifestyle modifications. It is important to talk to a healthcare provider about the best treatment plan for an individual's specific needs.

Overall, understanding obesity is essential in order to prevent and manage it. By making lifestyle changes and engaging in regular physical activity, individuals can reduce their risk of obesity and its associated health consequences.

Definition of Obesity

Obesity is a medical condition in which excess body fat has built up to the extent that it may have a negative effect on health. It is generally defined by an adult's body mass index (BMI) , a measure of weight relative to height that is greater than 30.

Causes And Contributing Factors Of Obesity

Causes Of Obesity

- Unhealthy diet

Eating high-calorie foods and not getting enough exercise can lead to weight gain and obesity. Eating fast food, processed foods, and sugary drinks are common culprits.

- Lack of physical activity

People who do not engage in enough physical activity are more likely to gain weight. This includes children who sit in front of screens for long periods of time.

- Genetics

Genetics can play a role in obesity. Some people may be predisposed to gaining weight more easily than others.

- Medications

Certain medications can cause people to gain weight. These include some steroids, antidepressants, and antipsychotics.

- Stress

Stress can result in eating too much and weight gain.

- Sleep deprivation

People who deprive themselves of sleep may be more likely to gain weight.

- Hormonal imbalances

Hormonal imbalances, such as hypothyroidism, can cause people to gain weight.

Contributing Factors of Obesity

- Lack of access to healthy food

People who live in areas with limited access to healthy food may be more likely to gain weight.

- Socioeconomic status

People who have lower socioeconomic status may be more likely to gain weight due to limited access to healthy food, lack of education, and higher stress levels.

- Certain medical conditions

Some diseases and illnesses such as polycystic ovary syndrome (PCOS), can cause you to gain weight.

- Certain medications

Certain medications, such as corticosteroids and some antidepressants, can cause people to gain weight.

- Age

Ageing is a factor for weight gain. As we grow our metabolism slows down, which can lead to weight gain.

- Lack of education

People who do not have enough education about nutrition, exercise, and healthy habits may be more likely to gain weight.

- Social environment

People who lack social support or who are exposed to negative influences may be more likely to gain weight.

Health Risks And Complications Of Obesity

Obesity is a serious health condition that can lead to a number of health risks and complications. Obese individuals have a higher risk of developing a variety of diseases, such as type 2 diabetes, heart disease, stroke, certain types of cancer, and other chronic diseases. They are also at a higher risk for developing sleep apnea, high blood pressure, high cholesterol, and fatty liver disease. Additionally, obesity can lead to issues with mental health, such as depression, low self-esteem, and increased stress. Obesity can also lead to physical complications, such as joint pain, difficulty breathing, and fatigue. Some people may also experience skin problems, such as stretch marks and skin infections. Obese individuals are also more likely to suffer from infertility, menstrual irregularities, and miscarriages. Finally, obese individuals may experience social stigmas related to their weight, which can lead to discrimination and isolation. This can be detrimental to a person's mental health and well-being. If you are obese, it is important to take action to reduce your risk of developing health complications. This includes following a healthy diet, exercising regularly, and maintaining a healthy weight. Additionally, it is important to speak to your doctor about any health risks and complications you get.

Chapter 2

Healthy Eating and Nutrition

Healthy eating and nutrition are essential for a healthy and balanced lifestyle. Healthy eating includes choosing a variety of foods from all the food groups and limiting the intake of unhealthy foods. Eating healthy can provide your body with the vitamins, minerals, and nutrients it needs to function properly and stay healthy.

Good nutrition is important for everyone, regardless of age, gender, or lifestyle. Eating a balanced diet can help you maintain a healthy weight, reduce your risk of chronic diseases such as diabetes and heart disease, and even help you look and feel better.

To get the most out of your meals, eat a variety of foods from each food group. Include plenty of fruits and vegetables, whole grains, low-fat dairy products, and lean proteins. Reduce your consumption of processed foods, saturated fats, and added sugars.

Eating healthy also involves being mindful of the portion sizes of the foods you eat. Eating too much or too little can lead to weight gain or health issues. It's important to listen to your body and only eat when you're hungry and stop when you're full.

Finally, staying hydrated is also essential for good health. Try as much as possible to drink plenty of water all through the day to stay hydrated and to help your body function properly.

By following these healthy eating and nutrition guidelines, you can maintain a healthy lifestyle and reduce your risk of developing chronic diseases. Eating healthy can also help you look and feel great, so it's worth the effort!

Eating Healthy

Eating healthy is an essential part of living a healthy lifestyle. Eating a balanced diet that includes fruits, vegetables, whole grains, and lean proteins can help you maintain a healthy weight, get the nutrients your body needs, and reduce your risk for certain chronic diseases.

To start eating healthy, it is important to understand the basics of nutrition. Learn which foods are high in certain vitamins and minerals and which foods should be limited or avoided. Focus on eating a variety of whole, unprocessed foods to get the most nutritional value.

In addition to eating a healthy diet, it is important to establish healthy eating habits. Try to aim for three meals a day and space them out evenly. Eat slowly and take breaks in between bites to give your body time to register when it is full. Also, try to avoid eating late at night or while distracted by activities such as watching television.

Eating healthy does not have to be boring. Experiment with new recipes, try new ingredients, and look for healthier alternatives to your favorite foods. Incorporating healthy snacks into your diet can also help keep you full and energized throughout the day. Eating healthy does not happen overnight. It takes time and effort to change your eating habits, but the rewards are worth it. Eating healthy can help you look and feel your best and reduce your risk for certain chronic conditions.

Nutrient-Dense Foods

Nutrient-dense foods are foods that are high in essential vitamins and minerals while being relatively low in calories. Examples of nutrient-dense foods include fruits and vegetables, lean meats, nuts and seeds, legumes, and whole grains. These foods provide essential vitamins and minerals, including antioxidants, polyphenols, and essential fatty acids, as well as fiber, which can help to support a healthy weight, reduce risk of chronic diseases, and promote overall health. Eating a variety of nutrient-dense foods can also help to ensure that you get enough of all the essential vitamins and minerals you need from your diet.

Meal Planning

Meal planning is a great way to save time, money, and stress when it comes to deciding what to eat. It involves deciding what meals to make ahead of time, and then shopping and prepping the ingredients in advance. Meal planning can help you stay organized, save money by buying in bulk, and reduce the risk of wasting food. It can also help you stick to a healthy eating plan, and make sure you are getting all the nutrients you need.

When meal planning, it's important to start by writing down your weekly meals, and then creating a grocery list based on what you need to make them. It's also important to consider food preferences, dietary restrictions, and any special occasions that might require a special meal. Additionally, it's important to think ahead and plan meals that use up fresh ingredients you already have in your fridge.

Once you have planned out your meals, it's time to shop. Many people prefer to shop online to save time, but if you can, try to shop at the store to get a better sense of what is available and on sale. When shopping, it's also a good idea to buy in bulk to save money, and to look for items that can be used in several different meals.

Finally, when you get home, it's important to prep your ingredients. This can include washing, chopping, marinating, and freezing ingredients ahead of time, so that when it's time to cook, everything is ready to go.

Meal planning can be a great way to save time and money, and to make sure you're eating healthy, balanced meals. With a little bit of planning and preparation, you'll be able to enjoy delicious, nutritious meals all week long.

Chapter 3

Physical Activity

Physical activity is any form of movement that is done to maintain or improve health. This includes activities such as walking, running, cycling, swimming, playing sports, and engaging in physical activities such as yoga or Pilates. Physical activity is important for overall health and well-being, and it can help reduce the risk of many chronic diseases, including heart disease, diabetes, and some cancers. Regular physical activity can also help to improve mood, sleep quality, and energy levels. It can also aid in reducing stress, anxiety, and depression. To get the most benefit from physical activity, it is important to be active on most days of the week and to incorporate a variety of activities into your routine.

Exercise And Weight Loss

Exercise is one of the most important components of a successful weight loss program. Consistent physical activity can help you lose and maintain weight as well as improve your overall health. Exercise can help you burn calories, build muscle, and increase energy levels. When combined with a healthy diet, exercise can be an effective tool for losing weight.

When first starting an exercise program, it's important to set realistic goals and find an activity that you enjoy. Start with a few minutes of physical activity each day and gradually build up to 30 minutes or more. Choose activities that you enjoy, such as walking, jogging, swimming, biking, or dancing. If you have difficulty finding the motivation to exercise, try working out with a friend or joining a local gym.

It's also important to remember that diet is an important part of any weight loss program. To maximize the benefits of exercise, it's important to eat a balanced diet that is low in saturated fat, sugar, and calories. Eating plenty of fruits, vegetables, whole grains, lean proteins, and healthy fats can help you reach your weight loss goals.

In addition to diet and exercise, it's important to get enough sleep and practice stress-management techniques. All of these strategies can help you reach your weight loss goals and maintain a healthy lifestyle.

Types Of Exercise

- Aerobic Exercise

Activities such as jogging, swimming, cycling, and dancing that increase your heart rate and breathing rate for an extended period of time.

- Strength Training

Exercises such as weight lifting, resistance bands, and bodyweight exercises that use your own body weight or resistance to build muscle and strength.

- Flexibility and Mobility

Exercises Stretches and movements that increase your range of motion and help keep your joints and muscles healthy.

- Core Training

Exercises that focus on strengthening your abdominal and back muscles, as well as your glutes and hips.

- Balance Exercises

Movements that improve your coordination, stability, and posture.

- High-Intensity Interval Training (HIIT)

Short bursts of intense exercise followed by periods of rest or active recovery.

- Yoga

An exercise that combines physical postures, breathing techniques, and meditation.

Creating an Exercise Plan

- Set realistic goals

Before you can create an effective exercise plan, you need to set achievable goals. Consider your lifestyle, current fitness level, and any medical conditions that may affect how much exercise you can do. Make sure to set goals that are pragmatic and manageable.

- Identify activities

Decide which activities you want to include in your exercise plan. Consider your interests and preferences, and choose activities that you enjoy and will stick with.

- Schedule your workouts

Determine when and how often you will exercise. Make sure to plan enough time for your workouts to be effective and keep you motivated.

- Monitor your progress

Track your progress and adjust your exercise plan as needed. This can help ensure that you are making progress and staying on track with your goals.

- Have fun

Finally, don't forget to have fun when exercising. Exercise should be enjoyable not a chore. Make sure to add variety and challenge to your workouts to keep them fun and engaging.

Chapter 4

Weight Management Strategies

Weight management strategies focus on creating a healthy lifestyle rather than just attempting to lose weight. To manage your weight, focus on healthy eating, regular physical activity, and setting realistic goals.

- Healthy Eating

Eating healthy is one of the most important aspects of weight management. Work towards eating a balanced diet that includes plenty of fruits, vegetables, whole grains, and lean proteins. Keep away from processed foods and foods that are high in sugar and saturated fat.

- Regular Physical Activity

Regular physical activity is essential for weight management. Aim to get at least 30 minutes of moderate intensity activity most days of the week. This includes walking, jogging, swimming, or biking.

- Setting Realistic Goals

It is important to set realistic goals when it comes to weight management. Losing too much weight too quickly is not healthy and can lead to health problems. Set a realistic goal for yourself and work towards it gradually.

- Stress Management

Stress is a paramount agent in weight gain. Finding ways to manage stress, such as taking breaks, engaging in relaxation activities, or talking to a friend, can help you maintain a healthy weight.

- Sleep

Getting enough sleep is important for weight management. Aim for at least 7-8 hours of sleep each night to help regulate hormones and maintain a healthy weight.

- Portion Control

Controlling the amount of food you eat is an important aspect of weight management. Pay attention to portion sizes when eating and opt for smaller servings. By following these strategies, you can create a healthy lifestyle and maintain a healthy weight.

Healthy Habits

- Exercise regularly

Aim for at least 30 minutes of physical activity, five days a week.

- Eat a balanced di

Endeavour to eat plenty of fruits, vegetables, lean proteins, and whole grains.

- Get enough sleep

Sleep for seven to eight hours of sleep each night.

- Practice mindfulness

Take some time each day to be mindful and focus on your breath, body, and surroundings.

- Drink plenty of water

Staying hydrated is key to good health.

- Stay active

Find ways to stay active throughout the day, such as taking the stairs instead of the elevator or walking to work.

- Avoid smoking

Smoking is bad for your health, and quitting can help you live longer.

- Manage stress

Take time each day to relax and de-stress.

- Maintain social connections

Keep in touch with family and friends, and seek out support when needed.

- Practice good hygiene

Wash your hands often, brush your teeth twice a day, and shower regularly.

- Set a realistic goal

Make sure to set a goal that is achievable and within your means. It is important to set a realistic goal that you are able to commit to and not something that you will be unable to complete.

- Keep track of your progress

Keeping track of your progress helps to motivate you and keeps you on track.

- Make a plan and stick to it.

Make sure to create a plan that you can stick to. Take into account what you eat, when you exercise, and any other factors that can help you reach your goal.

- Don't give up.

No matter how hard it seems, don't give up on your goal. Stay focused and determined and you will reach your goal in time.

- Celebrate your successes.

Celebrate each small victory and make sure to reward yourself for your hard work. This will help to keep you inspired and focused.

Establishing Support Systems

Establishing support systems can be an important part of creating a healthy and successful environment. Support systems are tools and resources that can help individuals make sense of their environment, understand their choices, and make positive decisions. They can come in many forms, such as close friends, family, mentors, counsellors, and professional organizations.When establishing support systems, it is important to create an environment that is conducive to growth and development. This can be accomplished by providing resources such as education, mentorship, and support networks. Additionally, it is important to ensure that individuals are given the opportunity to express their feelings, thoughts, and opinions in a safe and supportive environment.

It is also important to ensure that individuals have access to resources, such as mental health services, financial assistance, and employment opportunities. These resources can help individuals build confidence and create positive outcomes. Additionally, it is important to ensure that individuals have access to support networks that provide support and guidance.

Finally, it is important to ensure that individuals are able to build meaningful relationships with those around them. This can be done by providing opportunities to socialize, engaging in activities together, and encouraging open communication.

By establishing support systems and providing individuals with the necessary resources and support, it is possible to create an environment in which individuals can thrive and reach their fullest potential.

Chapter 5

Recipes

Breakfast

Breakfast

- **Banana Oatmeal Pancakes**

Ingredients

- 2 medium-sized ripe bananas, mashed
- 2 eggs
- 1/4 cup almond milk
- 1/2 teaspoon vanilla extract
- 1/2 cup rolled oats
- 1/2 teaspoon baking powder
- 1 teaspoon cinnamon
- Pinch of salt
- Coconut oil or butter, for cooking

Instructions

1. In a medium bowl, mash the bananas until they are almost smooth.

2. Add the eggs, almond milk, and vanilla extract and mix until combined.
3. Add the oats, baking powder, cinnamon, and salt and mix until combined.

4. Heat a skillet over medium-high heat and add a teaspoon of coconut oil or butter.

5. Scoop a spoonful of the batter onto the pan and spread it out into a pancake shape.

6. Cook for about 3-4 minutes on each side, until golden brown.

7. Serve with your favorite toppings and enjoy!

- **Egg and Avocado Toast**

Ingredients:
- 2 slices of whole wheat bread
- 1 ripe avocado
- 2 eggs

- Salt and pepper to taste

Instructions:
1. Preheat the oven to 400°F.
2. Toast the bread in the oven for 5-7 minutes.
3. Peel and mash the avocado in a bowl.
4. In a separate bowl, beat the eggs and season with salt and pepper.
5. Heat a non-stick pan over medium-high heat.
6. Add the eggs to the pan and scramble.
7. Once the eggs are cooked, spread the mashed avocado on the toast.
8. Top with the scrambled eggs.
9. Enjoy!

- **Overnight Oats**

Ingredients:

-1/2 cup of old-fashioned rolled oats
-1/2 cup of your favorite milk
-3 tablespoons of chia seeds
-1/2 teaspoon of ground cinnamon
-A pinch of sea salt

-1 tablespoon of pure maple syrup
-1/2 cup of fresh or frozen fruit of your choice

Instructions:

1. In a medium-sized bowl, stir together the oats, chia seeds, cinnamon, and salt.

2. Pour in the milk and maple syrup and mix until everything is combined.

3. Add the fruit of your choice and stir again.

4. Cover the bowl and place it in the refrigerator overnight.

5. In the morning, give the oats a stir and enjoy!

Sweet Potato Toast recipe

Ingredients:

-1 large sweet potato, washed
-1 tablespoon olive oil
-Salt and pepper, to taste
-Toppings of your choice

Instructions:

1. Preheat the oven to 400°F (200°C).

2. Slice the sweet potato into 1/4-inch-thick slices.

3. Place the slices on a baking sheet lined with parchment paper.

4. Brush the slices with olive oil and season with salt and pepper.

5. Bake for 15 minutes, then flip the slices and bake for another 10 minutes, or until the slices are golden and crispy.

6. Once the slices are ready, let them cool for a few minutes before topping with your favorite toppings. Enjoy!

- **Greek Yogurt Parfait**

Ingredients:

-1 cup Greek yogurt

-½ cup fresh or frozen berries
-2 tablespoons honey
-2 tablespoons chopped almonds
-2 tablespoons granola

Instructions:

1. In a medium bowl, mix together the yogurt, berries and honey.

2. Place the yogurt mixture into a parfait glass or bowl.

3. Top with the chopped almonds and granola.

4. Serve and enjoy!

LUNCH

- **Grilled Chicken and Vegetable Salad**

Ingredients:
- 2 chicken breasts
- 2 tablespoons olive oil
- 1/2 teaspoon garlic powder

- 1/2 teaspoon oregano
- 1/2 teaspoon salt
- 1/4 teaspoon black pepper
- 2 tablespoons balsamic vinegar
- 2 cups chopped romaine lettuce
- 1/2 cup cherry tomatoes
- 1/2 red bell pepper, chopped
- 1/4 cup sliced red onion
- 1/4 cup sliced cucumber
- 2 tablespoons feta cheese

Instructions:
1. Preheat a grill or grill pan over medium-high heat.
2. In a bowl, combine the olive oil, garlic powder, oregano, salt, and pepper. Rub the chicken breasts with the oil mixture.
3. Grill the chicken for about 5 minutes on each side, or until cooked through.
4. To assemble the salad, combine the romaine, tomatoes, bell pepper, red onion, and cucumber in a large bowl.
5. Drizzle with the balsamic vinegar and toss to coat.

6. Top with the grilled chicken and feta cheese.

7. Serve and enjoy!

- **Veggie Quinoa Bowl**

Ingredients:

-1 cup cooked quinoa

-1/2 cup cooked sweet potato cubes

-1/2 cup cooked chickpeas

-1/2 cup cooked broccoli florets

-1/4 cup chopped red onion

-1/4 cup diced red bell pepper

-2 tablespoons olive oil

-1 teaspoon garlic powder

-1 teaspoon smoked paprika

-Salt and pepper, to taste

Instructions:

1. Preheat the oven to 400°F.

2. Spread sweet potato cubes, chickpeas, and broccoli onto a baking sheet. Drizzle with olive

oil, garlic powder, smoked paprika, and salt and pepper. Toss to coat.

3. Bake for 25 minutes, stirring halfway through.

4. Meanwhile, cook quinoa according to package instructions.

5. Once quinoa and roasted veggies are done cooking, combine in a large bowl with chopped red onion and red bell pepper.

6. Serve warm and enjoy!

- **Veggie Wraps**

Ingredients

- 2 whole-wheat wraps
- 2 tablespoons hummus
- 1/2 cup cooked quinoa
- 1/2 cup shredded carrots
- 1/2 cup shredded cabbage
- 1/4 cup diced red onion

- 1/4 cup diced bell pepper
- 1/4 cup sliced cucumber
- 2 tablespoons fresh parsley
- 2 tablespoons olive oil
- Salt and pepper to taste

Instructions

1. In a medium bowl, combine quinoa, carrots, cabbage, onion, bell pepper, and cucumber.

2. Drizzle with olive oil and season with salt and pepper.

3. Lay out the wraps and spread each one with a tablespoon of hummus.

4. Divide the veggie mixture between the two wraps, top with parsley, and roll up.

- **Grilled Chicken and Veggie Skewers**

Ingredients:

-1 lb boneless, skinless chicken breasts, cut into cubes
-2 bell peppers, cut into 1-inch cubes
-1 large red onion, cut into 1-inch cubes
-1 zucchini, cut into 1-inch cubes
-2 tablespoons olive oil
-1 teaspoon garlic powder
-1 teaspoon dried oregano
-1 teaspoon smoked paprika
-Salt and pepper, to taste

Instructions:

1. Preheat a grill or grill pan to medium heat.

2. In a large bowl, combine the chicken, bell peppers, red onion, zucchini, olive oil, garlic powder, oregano, smoked paprika, salt, and pepper. Toss to combine.

3. Thread the chicken and vegetables onto metal or wooden skewers.

4. Place the skewers on the preheated grill and cook for 8-10 minutes, flipping once and brushing with additional olive oil, if needed.

5. Serve with a side salad or other favorite side dish. Enjoy!

- **Grilled Chicken, Sweet Potato and Broccoli Bowl**

Ingredients:

- 2 boneless, skinless chicken breasts
- 1 large sweet potato, cubed
- 2 cups of broccoli florets
- 2 tablespoons olive oil
- Salt and pepper to taste

Instructions:

1. Preheat the oven to 375 degrees F.

2. Place chicken breasts on a baking sheet. Drizzle with 1 tablespoon of olive oil, and season with salt and pepper. Bake for 20 minutes or until cooked through.

3. Meanwhile, place cubed sweet potatoes on a separate baking sheet. Drizzle with 1 tablespoon of olive oil and season with salt and pepper. Bake for 25 minutes or until tender.

4. In a large skillet, heat remaining olive oil over medium heat. Add broccoli florets and season with salt and pepper. Cook for 5 minutes or until broccoli is tender.

5. To assemble, divide chicken, sweet potato, and broccoli between two bowls. Enjoy!

DINNER

- **Grilled Salmon with Avocado Salsa recipe**

Ingredients

- 2 salmon fillets
- 2 tablespoons olive oil
- Salt and pepper to taste

For the Avocado Salsa
- 1 ripe avocado, diced
- 1/2 cup diced tomatoes
- 1/4 cup diced red onion
- 1 jalapeno, seeded and diced
- 2 tablespoons chopped fresh cilantro
- Juice of 1 lime
- Salt and pepper to taste

Instructions

1. Preheat a grill or grill pan to medium-high heat.

2. Brush each salmon fillet with olive oil and season with salt and pepper.

3. Grill the salmon for 4-5 minutes per side, or until the salmon is cooked through.

4. While the salmon is cooking, prepare the avocado salsa by combining all the ingredients in a bowl and stirring until combined.

5. Serve the salmon topped with the avocado salsa. Enjoy!

- **Vegetarian Chilli**

Ingredients

- 2 tablespoons olive oil
- 1 large onion, diced
- 2 bell peppers, diced
- 2 cloves garlic, minced
- 2 jalapeños, seeded and minced
- 2 tablespoons chili powder
- 2 teaspoons cumin
- 1 teaspoon smoked paprika
- 1 teaspoon oregano
- 1/4 teaspoon cayenne pepper

- 2 (14.5-ounce) cans diced tomatoes
- 1 (15-ounce) can kidney beans, drained and rinsed
- 1 (15-ounce) can black beans, drained and rinsed
- 1 (15-ounce) can pinto beans, drained and rinsed
- 1 (15-ounce) can corn, drained and rinsed
- 2 cups vegetable broth
- 1/2 teaspoon salt
- 1/4 teaspoon black pepper
- 2 tablespoons lime juice
- Optional toppings: diced avocado, jalapeños, sour cream, shredded cheese, diced red onion, cilantro

Instructions

1. Heat the oil in a large pot over medium heat.

2. Add the onion, bell peppers, garlic, and jalapeños, and sauté for 5 minutes.

3. Add the chilli powder, cumin, smoked paprika, oregano, and cayenne pepper, and sauté for 1 minute.

4. Add the diced tomatoes, kidney beans, black beans, pinto beans, corn, vegetable broth, salt, and pepper. Bring to a boil, reduce heat to low, and simmer, uncovered, for 30 minutes, stirring occasionally.

5. Stir in the lime juice.

6. Serve with desired toppings. Enjoy!

- **Turkey and Spinach Meatballs**

Ingredients:

-1 lb ground turkey
-1/2 cup diced onion

-1/2 cup diced celery

-1/4 cup diced fresh garlic

-1/4 cup diced red bell pepper

-2 tablespoons olive oil

-1 cup fresh spinach, chopped

-1/2 cup bread crumbs

-1 egg

-2 tablespoons Italian seasoning

-1 teaspoon salt

-1/2 teaspoon black pepper

-1/4 cup grated Parmesan cheese

Instructions:

1. Preheat the oven to 375°F.

2. In a large skillet, heat olive oil over medium heat. Add onion, celery, garlic, and bell pepper. Cook until vegetables are tender, about 5 minutes.

3. Remove from heat and add spinach. Stir until spinach is wilted. Allow to cool.

4. In a large bowl, combine ground turkey, bread crumbs, egg, Italian seasoning, salt, pepper, Parmesan cheese, and cooled vegetable mixture. Mix until all ingredients are evenly combined.

5. Form mixture into 1-inch balls. Place on a greased baking sheet.

6. Bake in a preheated oven for 15-20 minutes, or until cooked through.

7. Serve with your favorite sauce or over pasta. Enjoy!

- **Roasted Vegetable Quinoa Bowl**

Ingredients:

- 2 cups cooked quinoa
- 2 cups assorted vegetables, such as bell peppers, zucchini, mushrooms, and red onion, chopped
- 2 tablespoons olive oil

- 1 teaspoon garlic powder
- 1 teaspoon dried oregano
- Salt and pepper to taste
- ½ cup feta cheese, crumbled
- 2 tablespoons fresh parsley, chopped

Instructions:

1. Preheat the oven to 400°F.
2. Spread vegetables out on a baking sheet. Drizzle with olive oil, garlic powder, oregano, salt, and pepper. Toss to combine.

3. Roast vegetables for 25-30 minutes, stirring once or twice, until vegetables are tender and lightly browned.
4. Divide cooked quinoa among four bowls. Top with roasted vegetables and feta cheese.

5. Garnish with parsley and serve.

- **Kale and Mushroom Quinoa**

Ingredients:

- 1 cup dry quinoa
- 1 tablespoon olive oil
- 1/2 cup diced onion
- 2 cloves garlic, minced
- 1/2 cup sliced mushrooms
- 1/2 cup diced kale
- 1/4 teaspoon each of sea salt and black pepper
- 2 cups vegetable broth

Instructions:

1. Rinse quinoa in a fine mesh strainer and set aside.

2. Heat olive oil in a large saucepan over medium heat. Add the onions and garlic and sauté until softened, about 5 minutes.

3. Add the mushrooms and kale and sauté for another 5 minutes.

4. Add the quinoa and season with sea salt and black pepper. Stir to combine and cook for another 2 minutes.

5. Pour in the vegetable broth, bring to a boil, reduce heat to low, cover and simmer for 20 minutes.

6. Remove from heat and let stand for 5 minutes. Fluff with a fork and serve. Enjoy!

SNACKS

- **Edamame**

Ingredients:

-1 pound of shelled edamame
-2 tablespoons of olive oil
-1 teaspoon of garlic powder
-1 teaspoon of onion powder
-Salt and pepper, to taste

Instructions:

1. Preheat oven to 400 degrees Fahrenheit.

2. Place edamame in a large bowl.

3. Drizzle olive oil over edamame and sprinkle with garlic powder, onion powder, salt, and pepper.

4. Use your hands to mix everything together until edamame is evenly coated.

5. Spread edamame onto a baking sheet and bake for 20 minutes, stirring once halfway through.

6. Enjoy your edamame warm!

- **Greek Yogurt with Berries**

Ingredients:

-2 cups of Greek yogurt

-1/2 cup of fresh or frozen berries of your choice
-1/4 cup honey
-1/4 cup of toasted nuts (optional)

Instructions:

1. In a medium bowl, combine the yogurt, berries, and honey. Stir until evenly combined.

2. Divide the yogurt mixture into two serving bowls.

3. Sprinkle the toasted nuts on top of the yogurt mixture.

4. Serve and enjoy!

- Hummus and Veggies recipe

Ingredients:

-1 can of chickpeas

-4 tablespoons of tahini
-4 tablespoons of lemon juice
-2 cloves of garlic
-1/4 teaspoon of ground cumin
-1/2 teaspoon of sea salt
-2 tablespoons of olive oil
-1/4 cup of water
-Assorted vegetables of your choice

Instructions:

1. Drain and rinse the chickpeas.

2. Place the chickpeas, tahini, lemon juice, garlic, cumin, salt, and olive oil in a food processor and blend until smooth.

3. Add the water, 1 tablespoon at a time, until desired consistency is reached.

4. Spread the hummus in a shallow dish or plate.

5. Chop the vegetables of your choice and arrange them around the hummus.

6. Serve and enjoy!

- **Trail Mix**

Trail mix is a snack food typically made of a combination of nuts, dried fruit, and other small snacks. It is great for eating on the go, giving you sustained energy and a nutritious snack. It is also very easy to make your own trail mix, so you can customize it to your own tastes and preferences. Common ingredients in trail mix include raisins, peanuts, almonds, cashews, sunflower seeds, pumpkin seeds, dried cranberries, and chocolate chips.

- **Avocado Toast recipe**

Ingredients:

- 2 slices of whole wheat or multigrain bread
- 1 ripe avocado

- 1 tablespoon of lemon juice
- ¼ teaspoon of garlic powder
- ¼ teaspoon of salt
- 2 teaspoons of olive oil
- 2 tablespoons of crumbled feta cheese
- Freshly ground black pepper
- Freshly chopped parsley (optional)

Instructions:
1. Toast the bread slices in a toaster or in a skillet.

2. Cut the avocado in half, remove the pit and scoop out the flesh with a spoon. Place the avocado in a bowl and mash it with a fork.

3. Add the lemon juice, garlic powder, salt, olive oil and mix everything together until a creamy texture is formed.
4. Spread the mashed avocado onto the toasted bread slices.
5. Sprinkle the crumbled feta cheese on top and season with freshly ground black pepper.

6. Garnish with freshly chopped parsley (optional).

7. Serve and enjoy!

Conclusion

The weight loss cookbook is a fantastic tool to help you reach your weight loss goals. With its simple and delicious recipes, you can easily incorporate healthy eating habits into your lifestyle. And with its practical tips and guidance, you can be sure to stay on track with your weight loss journey. So, if you're looking for a comprehensive and easy-to-follow guide to losing weight, the weight loss cookbook is the perfect choice. With its help, you can make healthy and delicious meals that you'll enjoy and that will help you stay on track to achieving your health and wellness goals.